Cannabinoids And Terpenes

The Medicinal Benefits of Cannabis

By Ryder Management Inc

Copyright 2014 by Ryder Management Inc
All Rights Reserved

ISBN: 1502597713

Prologue

"We move forward and become like that which we think about. Isn't it time we began to think about what we're thinking about?"

Don Coyhis, Mohican, 1993

"An agreement made with the government is like the agreement a buffalo makes with the hunter after it has been pierced by many arrows. All it can do is lie down and give in."

Chief Ouray, Utel, C, 1868

"A man was chief only as long as he did the will of the people. If he got to be too chiefy, he'd go to sleep one night, and wake up the next morning to find that he was chief all to himself. The tribe would move away in the night, and they didn't wait four years to do it either."

Sun Bear, Chippewa, 1970

"And that, I guess, is what it all boils down to: do the right thing, everything goes fine; do the wrong thing, everything's a mess."

Robert Spott, Yurok, 1890

Ryder Management Inc

Table of Contents

Introduction 1

Indica 3

Purple Skunk 3

Taxonomy and Cultivation of Indica 4

Sativa vs. Indica 5

Cannabis and the US Pharmacopeia 6

Extracted from the 1936 11th edition of the US Pharmacopeia 6

Science is Prone to Manipulation 7

Testing the Potency of Cannabis at Home 9

Gas Chromatography 11

High Performance Liquid Chromatography 12

Thin Layer Chromatography (TLC) 13

TLC – A Qualitative Method for Identifying Cannabinoids 15

The Relationship of Cannabinoids 17

The Importance of Terpenes 19

Terpenes in Cannabis 21

Therapeutic Benefits of Cannabinoids 24

Conclusion 25

Sample Lab Analysis Reports 26

Know Your Terpenes 28

Other Books by RMI 29

Ryder Management Inc

Introduction

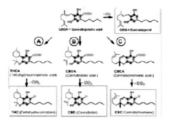

Although cannabis has been used as medicine for thousands of years throughout history, scientific information on cannabis has only recently been disclosed and made available to the masses. Previously, an elite group of individuals behind the United Nations and various government levels worldwide have falsely claimed some type of danger associated with cannabis use. Although we are now learning that although cannabis was included in the list of Controlled Drugs and Substances, the government in the US and UK have been privately conducting research and submitting applications for patents on the medical use of cannabis for as long as it has been criminalized. However absurd it may be, cannabis was considered a drug that had "no accepted medical use in treatment; no accepted safety use even under medical supervision" and was considered a drug "with a high potential for abuse", and for these reasons, was classified under Schedule I at the time the "Controlled Drugs and Substances Act" came into force in the early seventies.

This book includes information on two important organic compounds found in the cannabis plant, namely cannabinoids and terpenes. Cannabinoids and terpenes are considered "secondary plant metabolites" which means that although they don't play a part in the plant's primary metabolic requirements that involve the normal growth, development or reproduction of the plant, rather these compounds increase the plant's overall ability to survive and thrive. Cannabinoids are closely related "terpenophenolic" compounds which are natural products of mixed biosynthetic origin and specifically, they are a combination of hydrocarbon and carbonic acid molecules. (The above picture is an example of this). Terpenophenolic compounds also contain biological activities that make them important for human health.

Terpenes are a large and diverse class of organic compounds produced by a number of plants of which many are "aromatic hydrocarbons" (sometimes called arenes). When terpenes are chemically modified such as by oxidation, they are referred to as terpenoids. Terpenoids are also known as isoprenoids. Terpenes and terpenoids are the primary constituents of the essential oils of many plants including cannabis.

The synergistic effects of cannabinoids and terpenes offer a great deal of additional benefits which is only beginning to be investigated scientifically. As patients become more educated on the full potential of cannabis, cannabis preparations and with the complexities in the various compounds found within cannabis, they will become more discerning in choosing their medicine which will help increase the quality of the medication available to them along with the research relating to the synergistic benefits of cannabinoids and terpenes.

Indica

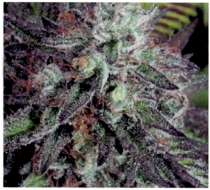

Purple Kush

As a connoisseur of cannabis, I am partial to the Indica species. I prefer strains in which her terpenes produce a sweet **skunk** smell and her trichomes are really sticky to the touch. Indica adapts and grows quite easily in potted containers. Relative to Sativa, Indica is short and stout and have fatter colas as harvest approaches. The crystal trichomes are also more noticeable and pronounced. The trichomes or crystals are where terpenes are produced and which give rise to that wonderful and distinct skunky scent many love. Some Indica strains have leaves with a purple tinge such as Purple Kush, pictured above, and Purple Skunk, below.

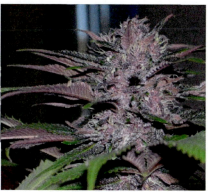

Purple Skunk

Other notable Indica dominant strains that are sticky, sweet smelling and loaded with crystals include Afghani Dream, White Widow, and LA Confidential. LA Confidential's lineage is from Afghani and Kush and is 100% Indica. Also a descendent of Afghani crossed with an Indica dominant hybrid is White Widow. White Widow grows gorgeous fat buds which are also loaded with crystals as harvest nears. This strain seemed to dominate the cannabis scene for a number of years, a number of years ago.

Taxonomy and Cultivation of Indica

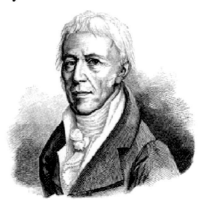

A description of "Cannabis Indica" was formally published in 1785 by a French naturalist, *"Jean-Baptiste Pierre Antoine de Monet, Chevalier de Lamarck"* pictured above. Jean-Baptist (August 1, 1744 – December 18, 1929) referred to this plant as "a second species of Cannabis" and called it *Cannabis Indica*, its binomial or scientific name that remains to this day. Jean-Baptiste, known as a French naturalist, was also a botanist, biologist, academic and soldier. As a botanist, Jean-Baptist studied and collected samples of plants. He named the Indica plant based on a species he had collected from India, *Cannabis Sativa (C. Sativa)*. Back in 1785, C. Indica was described as a short, densely branched bush whereas C. Sativa, her sister, was described as long and lanky. It was determined that Indica may have originated from the Hindu Kush mountain range, located between central Afghanistan and northern Pakistan. In the time of Alexander the Great, the Hindu Kush mountain range was referred to as *Caucasus Indicus*.

Indica **landraces** show a higher Cannabidiol (CBD) content relative to *Sativa*. A landrace is a term used to describe "a local variety of a domesticated plant species which has developed over time by adapting to the natural and cultural environment in which it lives". (*Wikipedia*)

Sativa vs. Indica

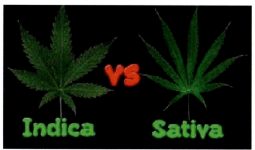

Compared to C. Sativa, C. Indica has more of a relaxed "stone" relative to the "high" associated with Sativa. Sativa, on the other hand, has been described more of a "spaced out" high that certain "stoners" tend to prefer. However, in terms of preference, there is probably an equal amount of proponents for both sides.

Due to the high quantity of Cannabidiol (CBD) in Indica, there is very little chance that this species will cause an anxiety or panic attack let alone, paranoia. Indica has an *anxiolytic* quality meaning that it has anti-panic and anti-anxiety qualities. (Anxiolytic inhibits anxiety whereas anxiogenic substances cause anxiety). Indica strains have a number of other beneficial qualities and are able to treat a great deal of ailments including insomnia and pain.

Sativas have much narrower leaves than Indicas and can reach heights of up to 20 feet, when conditions allow it. The leaves of Sativas are also known to be more of a lighter green, relative to the Indicas. Distinguishing between these two species can be quickly accomplished by looking at the leaves as can be noted in the picture above.

The cannabinoid CBD - Cannabidiol found in C. Indica is a 5-HT 1A receptor agonist. 5-HT 1A receptors are a subset of 5-HT serotonin receptors. Effects of the 5-HT 1A receptors that have been observed in scientific research include: decreased aggression, increased sociability, decreased impulsiveness, prolonged REM sleep, reversal of opioid induced respiratory depression and facilitation of sex drive and arousal. Activation of the 5-HT1A receptors has been involved in the "mechanism of action" in certain Psychopharmacology medications including anxiolytic, antidepressant and antipsychotic pills. This explains how smoking a joint can "take the edge off". With this information in mind, why do some from the scientific community claim that cannabis creates the very condition it helps?

Cannabis and the US Pharmacopeia

EXTRACTUM CANNABIS
Extract of Cannabis
Ext. Cannab.—Extractum Cannabis indicæ P.I.

Prepare an extract by percolating 1000 Gm. of cannabis, in moderately coarse powder, using alcohol as the menstruum. Macerate the drug during forty-eight hours and then percolate it at a moderate rate until the drug is exhausted. Evaporate the percolate to a pilular consistence at a temperature not exceeding 70° C., and mix the mass thoroughly.

AVERAGE DOSE—Metric, 0.015 Gm.—Apothecaries, ¼ grain.

Extracted from the 1936 11th edition of the US Pharmacopeia

The United States Pharmacopeia was founded in 1820. It is the U.S. Pharmacopeia Convention (USP) that has been set up as a non-profit organization and sets the "standards for the identity, strength quality and purity of medicines, food ingredients and dietary supplements manufactured, distributed and consumed worldwide." (usp.org)

In reviewing the fabulous information provided by "antiquecannabisbook.com" we learn that Cannabis was first listed in 1851 in the US Pharmacopoeia's Third Edition. We also learn that in 1851 there was little or no government interference and the Pharmacopeia's purpose was "to identify and standardize the then most botanical drugs in medicinal use".

Cannabis was listed in the U.S. Pharmacopeia continually from 1851 until the mid-thirties of the twentieth century when the US Federal Government "joined a campaign to outlaw medical cannabis in whatever form. The campaign, which made effective use of radio, magazine and newspaper articles, spoke of the evils of the medical Cannabis plant, that its use would lead to insanity, to the commission of the most depraved acts including rape, child molestation, axe murders, etc." (antiquecannabisbook.com)

Where cannabis was once as common as aspirin, the 12th edition of the U.S. Pharmacopeia 1942 was the last mention of the medical use of the Cannabis plant.

Science is Prone to Manipulation

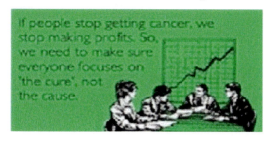

There exists a great deal of published research originating from 1975 to 1996 that is having a significant influence on "marijuana ballot initiatives".

From the International Drug Strategy Institute, Topeka, Kansa, University of Kansas School of Medicine, Kansas City Kansas, and Fairfax Hospital, Falls Church, Virginia, this author cites the following:

Marijuana has been widely used for hundreds of years as an intoxicant or herbal remedy. Pure delta- 9-tetrahydrocannabinol (THC) is the major active ingredient in marijuana and is 1 of 66 cannabinoid constituents of marijuana. It is now available by prescription as dronabinol. The use of crude marijuana as a medicine would entail smoking the drug or creating herbal preparations of it. Crude marijuana, an undefined herb containing approximately 480 substances (1) has not been approved by the U.S. Food and Drug Administration for use as medicine." Conclusions state that crude marijuana is unsafe.

The American Medical Association (AMA), in a published document states that they endorse "well controlled studies of marijuana and related cannabinoids in patients with serious conditions for which preclinical anecdotal, or controlled evidence suggests possible efficacy and the applications of such results to the understanding and treatment of disease.:" However, they continued to support marijuana's status as a Schedule 1 controlled substance. Then again in 2011, although they agreed to be in support of alternative delivery methods of cannabis they also stated that "this should not be viewed as an endorsement of state based medical cannabis programs, the legalization of marijuana, or that scientific evidence on the therapeutic use of cannabis meets the current standards for prescription drug product". For those unaware of the history of the AMA, further research would be in order.

The American Cancer Society (ACS) "does not advocate inhaling smoke, nor the legalization of marijuana" despite agreeing to support carefully controlled clinical studies for alternative delivery methods, specifically a tetrahydrocannabinol (THC) skin patch.

Continuing to list like-minded published reports from similar controlled organization's archives, is beyond the intended scope of this book. Suffice it to say, caution and a grain of salt is necessary when reading any information; regardless of whether it cites "scientific proof". Always ensure to do your own research.. After all, cannabis is and will remain a natural plant gifted from Mother Nature.

Testing the Potency of Cannabis at Home

Since using the Rick Simpson (hash) oil method (i.e. the RSO method for treating cancer), I was determined to find out exactly which cannabinoids were involved that saved me from the fate of chemo, radiation or an untimely demise. Since I had just begun to hear of "cannabis test kits" for the purpose of testing cannabinoids in cannabis strains, I began researching what was available and whether one existed for home use by a patient. To this end, the following describes Chromatography and the various methods available as they apply to the Medical Cannabis market. The focus however, was with finding one available for home use.

With the rise in Medical Marijuana Dispensaries came a demand for the ability to identify and quantify the cannabinoids in any given strain. Although dispensaries , collectives, growers and edible companies in the US and Licensed Producers in Canada are expected to test the cannabis they supply including disclosing this information to their buyers and patients, the buyers and patients whose need for cannabis is relatively small, should also have the ability to employ an inexpensive cannabinoid testing method at home.

At the core of this demand for testing, came enterprises marketing "novel testing kits". The variation in testing methods that have emerged can be categorized as follows: GC –Gas Chromatography, HPLC - High Performance Liquid Chromatography and HPTLC. High Performance Thin Layer Chromatograph, which is sometimes simply called TLC – Thin Layer Chromatography.

Chromatography is the "collective term for a set of laboratory techniques used in the separation of mixtures" (Wikipedia). Although there are basically three chromatography techniques that presently exist for testing a strain of cannabis, the methods differ in how the cannabinoids are separated. This can influence their ability to adequately qualify or quantify the cannabinoids being tested (distinguishing or determining the quantity).

The emerging Medical Marijuana industry is reported to be focusing a great deal of attention on the GC or the Gas Chromatography method, and due to aggressive marketing tactics, it is becoming the most common technique sold. "Gas Chromatography" it is said "is the economic standard within the Medicinal Marijuana arena".

All forms of chromatography involve a "stationary phase" and a "mobile phase". In the mobile phase, the sample is dissolved in a fluid which can be a liquid, however in Gas Chromatography (GC); the mobile phase involves a gas, such as helium. Normally the mobile phase carries the sample through a structure holding another substance and this part of testing is known as the stationary phase. In GC, this phase consists of a high boiling point liquid absorbed onto a solid.

Gas Chromatography

GAS CHROMATOGRAPHY

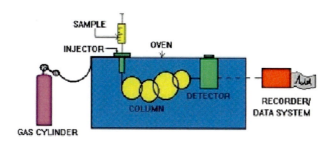

As previously stated, each method of chromatography involves a "stationary phase" and a "mobile phase". In Gas Chromatography, the mobile phase involves a gas, such as helium. The stationary phase is a high boiling point liquid absorbed onto a solid. Very small quantities of the sample being analyzed are injected into the machine using a small syringe. The column is packed with a finely ground "porous rock" which is coated with a high boiling liquid, typically a waxy polymer. This is the stationary phase. The temperature of the column can be varied but is typically lower than in the inject part of the oven.

The machine is expensively priced, as are the retail tests solicited to Dispensaries' and patients. This testing method takes a bud sample and using a vaporized method, it pushes the sample through a long thin tube that is coated with a mix of gases designed to separate the cannabinoids in that sample. The problem with this method is with the temperature at which decarboxylation takes place, and how this relates to not just the THC cannabinoid, but other cannabinoids including THCV, CBD, CBN, and CBG.

Unfortunately, due to the temperature at which decarboxylation takes place, the GC method is unable to properly distinguish between the various cannabinoids (qualify). More specifically, this method is unable to distinguish THC from THC-V or from CBDV, CBD, CBN and CBG. **However, this method is the cat's meow for those concerned with measuring just the THC content in their strain.** My requirement was ensuring my medicinal cannabis contained the level of CBD that I understood benefited my health condition the most.

High Performance Liquid Chromatography (HPLC)

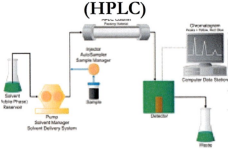

High Performance Liquid Chromatography (HPLC) is a form of column chromatography that is used frequently in analytical chemistry. To separate components in a test sample, this method uses a variety of chemical interactions between the compounds within the substance being tested and the chromatographic column. The parts that make up a basic High Performance Liquid Chromatography (HPLC) test method are shown in the above basic diagram.

With this method, a reservoir holds the solvent which is referred to as the mobile phase since it is the mover. The reservoir is shown on the above diagram on the left (holding the green solvent). The column container at the top of the above diagram represents the stationery phase. This column contains the chromatographic packing material needed to effect the separation. Since this packing material is held in place by the column hardware, this packing material is actually what represents the stationary phase in this example of a HPLC.

The detector is wired to a computer station and is the component that records the electrical signal needed to generate the chromatogram on its display and identify the constituents in a given sample. The detector uses ultraviolet lights as a detector.

In the HPLC or High Performance Liquid Chromatography testing method, the sample is also pushed through a short tube packed with silica particles by liquid solvents. The separated cannabinoids are measured at the far end, usually by using ultraviolet lights. Problems with this method include cross contamination, significant repairs and costly maintenance.

Thin Layer Chromatography (TLC)

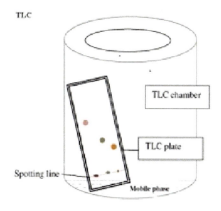

Thin layer chromatography (TLC) is a widely used chromatography technique used to separate specific components in a substance. The stationary phase consists of a thin layer of adsorbent material, usually silica gel on a flat inert carrier sheet, such as a piece of glass. The liquid or mobile phase consists of dissolving the material to be tested in an appropriate solvent. A sample is then drawn via capillary action separating the experimental solution. Although TLC can be configured for quantitative analysis, it is used mainly for qualitative analysis, in terms of identifying plant components.

Subsequent to researching GC and HPLC, I chose a simple TLC – Thin Layer Chromatography method of testing. The test kit I found was very inexpensive and included everything required to analyze samples of cannabis strains for cannabinoids, which I did shortly after harvest and curing. The TLC test kit is capable of analyzing bud samples for the presence of certain cannabinoids including THC, CBD, CBN and CBG. Although the Thin Layer Chromatography test kit I chose did not quantify the cannabinoids tested, rather, it was more of a qualitative technique to determine the relative presence of specific cannabinoids in a sample. However, the results could then be compared to a sample supplied containing specific quantitative lab results. This then allows one to determine the relative quantity of cannabinoids in any given sample.

The TLC method is capable of both Cold testing – which identifies cannabinoid acids (CBGA, THCA, CBDA, etc.) and Hot Testing - using a method of decarboxylation in order to test for THC, CBD CBG and CBN cannabinoids in a sample. Heating the samples does evaporate the CBD and CBN cannabinoids along with other substances that are known to evaporate at a lower temperature than THC does. This downfall however, also occurs in the previously discussed alternate methods of chromatography analysis too.

The Thin Layer Chromatography (TLC) method uses a piece of glass coated with a thin layer of solid adsorbent, silica. A small amount of the mixture to be analyzed is "spotted" near the bottom of the plate. In cold testing, this plate is placed immediately in a shallow pool of solvent (liquid) in a "developing chamber" so that the very bottom of the plate is submerged in the liquid (solvent). (The "developing chamber" was simply a glass jar in the TLC test kit I purchased.) The solvent or liquid fluid in the developing chamber is considered to be the **mobile phase** as it will slowly rise to the top of the plate by "capillary" action. As this solvent moves up the plate, it will carry the molecules in the cannabis samples. Once the solvent reaches the top of the plate, the plate is removed from the developing chamber and set aside to dry. Once the plate dries and sprayed with an identifying dye, the cannabinoids will become visible. This dye is specific to cannabinoids as each cannabinoid will be displayed in its own color, for example THC is red; CBC is yellow, CBD and CBG are both orange but in different locations and CBN are violet.

TLC – A Qualitative Method for Identifying Cannabinoids

Thin layer chromatography (TLC) is a technique used to determine the existence of specific cannabinoids that are present in medical cannabis. This technique is performed on a sheet of glass and through visual color indicators; one is able to determine whether the cannabis medicine contains specific cannabinoids including CBD, CBC CBG, THC and/ or cannabinoid groups.

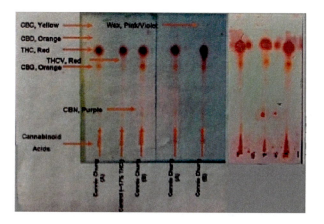

The picture above includes three glass plates with a thin layer of silica on the front. The left hand side was supplied with the test kit and is used as the controlled sample group to which those tests prepared at home can be compared to. The plate on the right hand side, are the test results from the three Indica strains I tested.

When this test was performed, I was quite shocked with these test results because I expected to see Cannabidiol (CBD). According to these test results, none of the three samples tested showed any existence of Cannabidiol (CBD). However, the test does identify the existence of CBG (Cannabigerol), as depicted by the orange dots directly below the larger red dots. The test shows the existence of THC as depicted by the large red dots, along with the identification of THCV, as depicted by the lighter red just below the red THC dots. There also seems to be the possible existence of CBN, if the color violet can be argued to exist on the lower part of the sample on the far right. All three strains tested were Indicas and the strains appear almost identical as depicted from the testing method chosen. It should be noted too that each strain tested was grown outdoors under protected conditions using only organic means and the test was performed shortly after each strain was harvested and cured. The strains, from left to right are: BC Bud; LA Confidential and a clone from an Indica Mother.

The testing method involved decarbing the samples (a.k.a. decarboxylation) by heating the thin layer chromatography (TLC) plate in a preheated oven at approximately 260 degrees for three to three and one half minutes prior to placing the plate directly into the "developing chamber". Prior to decarbing, the testing method involved "spotting" two microliters of each sample solution drawn from the stationery phase (in which the samples were contained in a separating solution) onto the TLC glass plate. I did find this part testing my patience while waiting for the drops. Therefore, the bleeding around the large red THC dots in the sample can be the result of my impatience. The results of the test also had me delve deeper into studying cannabinoids and other components of cannabis much further.

The Relationship of Cannabinoids

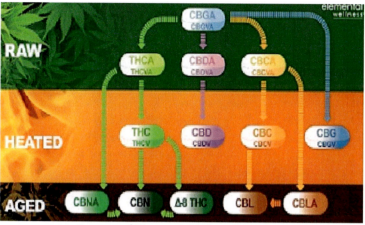

Courtesy of Elemental Wellness Dispensary

Cannabinoids are considered to be the main biologically active constituents in the cannabis plant and there are approximately 70 that have been identified, documented and described by science. In the past, very little information was made available on the CBG group of cannabinoids (the three main ones include CBG - Cannabigerol, CBGA -Cannabigerolic Acid and CBGV-Cannabigerivarin) since earlier studies focused mainly on the THC and CBD groups. Any mention of the CBG cannabinoid in the past reported that CBG existed mainly in the hemp plant. With the use of a thin layer chromatography test kit as a means of qualifying the cannabinoids present in my Indica strains, the result of the test revealed the presence of CBG but no CBD. Current publication from the scientific community now state that all cannabinoids, including THC, CBC CBD and CBG are derived from CBGA – Cannabigerolic Acid.

The above flowchart (from Elemental Wellness, a California Not-For-Profit) illustrates that (from enzymes within the cannabis plant); CBGA is converted to other cannabinoid acids including THCA - Tetrahydrocannabinolic Acid; CBDA - Cannabidiolic Acid and CBCA, Cannabichromic Acid. This shows that CBGA is the precursor to other cannabinoids and may also indicate that CBGV is a kind of stem cell for much of the medicinal effects within cannabis.

The above flow chart further illustrates that in its raw or unheated form, the cannabinoids CBGA and CBGVA are responsible for producing THCA and THCVA; ; CBDA and CBDVA; CBCA and CBCVA . It is not until these cannabinoids are heated and decarboxylation occurs that each of the aforementioned groups converts into THC, CBD, CBC and CBG. Decarboxylation is a chemical reaction that removes the carboxylic acids from the carbon chain (the A is removed).

Advances in laboratory analysis - have been made available to collectives and this has facilitated the understanding of medical cannabis on a deeper level. Much of the research currently underway is focused on being able to precisely describe the therapeutic effects of the cannabinoids and terpenoids within Cannabis. Two recent studies in this regard have been published by Izzo, et al (2009) and by Ethan Russo (2011).

Another key that helps us better understand medical cannabis is the awareness that the chemical compounds available in the plant change with the method of delivery. Potential benefits vary when administered or processed raw or unheated, heated and also when cannabis has degraded or aged.

It should also be noted that cannabinoids are known to also occur in certain other plant species besides cannabis. These include various species of Echinacea (E. purpurea, E, angustifolia and E. pallida), the jambu plant in Brazil known as Acmella, various species of Helichrysum brachyhynchum (related to the licorice plant) and Radula-marginata, a genus of liverworts. Radula is native to New Zealand and Tasmania.

The Importance of Terpenes

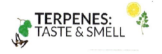

    Terpenes are a large and diverse class of naturally occurring organic compounds produced by a number of plants of which many are "aromatic hydrocarbons" (sometimes called arenes). When terpenes are chemically modified such as by oxidation, they are referred to as terpenoids. Terpenoids are also known as isoprenoids. Terpenes and terpenoids are the primary constituents of the essential oils of many plants and flowers including cannabis. The difference between terpenes and terpenoids is that terpenes are hydrocarbons whereas terpenoids contain "additional functional groups" (meaning they contain specific groups of atoms). Terpenes are volatile which means they can easily evaporate at normal temperatures or are liable to change quite rapidly and unpredictably, sometimes for the worse. They are the compounds in cannabis, as with other plants, that give rise to the plant's unique scent. Since cannabinoids have no smell, the unique scent within a cannabis strain is due to a unique combination of its terpenes.

    Terpenes are more volatile than cannabinoids and their presence relates to the freshness of the strain. It has long been known that therapeutic benefits can be had through aromatherapy, a form of alternative medicine that uses volatile plant materials and other aromatic compounds for health and other beneficial purposes. Therefore, just like the cannabinoids in cannabis, the terpenes in cannabis also produce many health benefits.

    Terpenes are referred to as terpenoids when they are denatured by oxidation such as when the cannabis plant has been dried and cured. Terpenes are also considered terpenoids when they have been chemically altered by some rearrangement of the carbon skeleton.

    There are approximately 120 known and distinct terpenes produced by the cannabis plant and the relative concentration of the individual terpenes varies considerably among the different strains of cannabis. Laboratory experiments have shown that it is impossible to recreate Cannabis resin to include the full medicinal effect that the cannabis plant is able to offer, by simply synthesizing some of the cannabinoids contained within cannabis.

From a chemical standpoint, terpenes are a large and varied class of hydrocarbons that make up a majority of plant resins and sap. The name terpene comes from "turpentine", which, in its raw form, is the sap from the Pine tree and which is terpene based. Essential oils are primarily composed of terpenes and have a very long history of use in medicine both topically and internally.

Terpenes are derived biosynthetically from units of isoprene (a colorless volatile liquid produced by many plants) with the molecular formula **C_5H_8**. The basic molecular formulae for terpenes are multiples of this basic formula or *(C_5H_8) n, where "n" is the number of isoprene units.* This is known as the C5 rule. The isoprene units can link "head to tail" to form linear chains or they can arrange themselves to form rings. An isoprene unit is considered one of Nature's common building blocks.

As isoprene units join together, the resulting terpenes are then classified according to sequential size. For example, a prefix to the terpene name is added to indicate the number of terpene units necessary to make up the molecule:

Hemiterpenes: a single isoprene unit

***Mono*terpenes:** two isoprene units with the molecular formula $C_{10}H_{16}$

***Sesqui*terpenes:** three isoprene units with the molecular formula $C_{15}H_{24}$

Bicyclic terpenes feature two fused rings.

Monoterpenes and sesquiterpenes are found to make up approximately 90% of the terpenes found in the cannabis plant.

Terpenes in Cannabis

Similar to other plants and flowers with a strong scent, terpenes in cannabis developed for a number of reasons including adaptive such as to repel predators and/or to lure pollinators. The resinous trichomes in the cannabis plant contain both the cannabinoids and the terpenes. A number of factors influence a cannabis strain's development of terpenes and include (but not limited to) atmosphere (whether grown indoors or outdoors), maturation, age, soil type and fertilizers. Some of the major terpenes found in various strains of Cannabis include:

Pinene: a montoterpene ($C_{10}H_{16}$) with a boiling point of 155C and with a pine aroma. In addition to cannabis, these terpenes are also found in the essential oils of many species of fur trees especially pine and also medicinal herbs including rosemary, basil, parsley, dill and the eucalyptus tree. Therapeutic benefits include antiseptic; expectorant; bronchodilator and as such can be a treatment for asthma; it also increases mental focus and energy. This terpene was found at the highest level in the Sativa strain Super Silver Haze when analyzed by the Green House Seed Company. Other strains these terpenes are found in include Jack Herer (Sativa), Chemdawg (Hybrid), Bubba Kush (Indica) and Trainwreck (Hybrid).

Borneol: bicyclic terpenes that are easily oxidized to the ketone yielding camphor with a boiling point of 213C. The scent can be described as menthol, pine, and woody. It is also easily converted into menthol. Borneol can also be found in cinnamon and wormwood, along with various strains of cannabis. Considered a calming sedative, its therapeutic benefits are analgesic, anti-insomnia, anti-septic and bronchodilator. It is also indicated for severe obstruction of the orifices, for heat syndromes, pain, and applied topically for a wide range of conditions. Borneol is also a natural insect repellent.

Carene: also called delta-3-carene, it is a bicyclic montoterpene ($C_{10}H_{16}$) with a boiling point of 169C. Carene also naturally occurs as a constituent of turpentine. Other sources include rosemary and cedar. Carene has a sweet and pungent odor that has been described as pine, cedar or woodsy like. It is said to be a central nervous system depressant. This terpene has been found in skunk varieties along with B 3985 TE and Amtbol 398 in high quantities both of which originate in Bolivia.

Beta-Caryophyllene (BCP): In addition to cannabis, this bicyclic sesquiterpene ($C_{15}H_{24}$) is also naturally found in basil, oregano, cinnamon bark, rosemary, hops , cloves and black pepper and contributes to the latter's spiciness. These terpenes have a boiling point of 130C. Therapeutic benefits include analgesic, anti-bacterial, anti-fungal, anti-inflammatory, bronchodilator and are effective at reducing neuropathic pain. This terpene also has gastro-protective qualities and is good for gastrointestinal complications. BCP also binds to the CB2 receptor, in fact, it acts specifically on the body's CB2 cannabinoid pathways and since CB2 is considered an endocannabinoid receptor (found in the body) BCP is being considered a cannabinoid. It is this scent that trainers teach drug dogs to find. Cannabis strains known to contain a high content of BCP include the Indica Hash Plant.

Cineole also called eucalyptol: described as spicy, refreshing, and minty. In addition to cannabis, these terpenes are also found in rosemary, sage, bay leaves, wormwood, tea tree, mugwort and eucalyptus. Therapeutic benefits include pain relief, increased circulation, anti-bacterial, anti-depressant, anti-inflammatory and bronchodilator.

Humulene: sesquiterpene ($C_{15}H_{24}$) with a boiling point of 107C. Besides cannabis, these terpenes are also found in pine trees, orange orchards, tobacco, sage, spearmint, ginger, Vietnamese coriander, hops basil and sunflowers. Humulene has anti-inflammatory effects and has the potential to be effective in managing autoimmune or inflammatory diseases. This terpene is also effective in treating conditions of edema and is anti-cancer. Strains that include a noticeable high quantity of Humulene include Skunk, Swissmix from Switzerland and Bolivia's Amtbol 398.

Limonene: C10H16 with a boiling point of 176C and a citrus aroma. These terpenes are also found in citrus fruit rinds, rosemary and juniper. Limonene is often repulsive to predators. It is a potent anti-fungal and anti-cancer agent. Other therapeutic benefits are anti-anxiety, anti-bacterial, anti-cancer, anti-depressant, bronchodilator and dissolving gallstones. Limonene is also thought to enhance alertness and focus attention; increased cerebral acetylcholine activity which decreases memory loss. This terpene is also commonly found in many strains of cannabis. This terpene is also used in chemical synthesis as a precursor to carvone and also used as a renewably based solvent in cleaning products. Hybrid strains with high limonene terpenes include OG Kush, Super Lemon Haze and Lemon Skunk.

Linalool: C10H18O with a boiling point of 198C. Its aroma is described as citrus, candy, floral scent similar to spring flowers. Linalool is found in over 200 species of plants mainly from the families Lamiaceae (mints); Lauraceae (laurels, cinnamon, and rosewood) and Rutaceae (citrus fruits). Therapeutic benefits include anti-stress, anti-anxiety, anti-bacterial, anti-convulsive, anti-depressant, anti-insomnia and effective in pain management. It is also useful as an anesthetic, anti-allergy and a Broncho relaxant. Linalool also has anti-anxiety properties and is used in the treatment of both psychosis and anxiety disorders plus it has been effectively used as an anti-epileptic agent. Linalool is also a very important precursor in the formation of Vitamin E. Strains with a high Linalool content include LA Confidential (Indica), Lavender (Hybrid) and G-13 (Indica).

Myrcene: a montoterpene (C10H16) with a boiling point of 167C. This scent is described as clove like, earthy, fruity with tropical mango and minty nuances. Myrcene is the most prevalent terpene found in most varieties of cannabis and it is also found in high amounts in lemongrass, mangos, hops, thyme, black pepper and verbena. It is a known building block for menthol, citronella and geraniol. Therapeutic benefits include analgesic, anti-cancer, anti-inflammatory, anti-insomnia and anti-spasmodic, anti-oxidant, antimicrobial, antiseptic, anti-depressant, anti-inflammatory and muscle relaxing effects. Myrcene is found in most strains of cannabis but not hemp. This terpene is found in various strains of cannabis including Pure Kush (Indica), Skunk #1 (Sativa) and El Nino (Hybrid).

Terpinolene: part of a group of terpenes from the group terpinenes. Terpinolene is also found in apples, cumin, lilac, tea tree and conifers. The scent is soft smoky, woody. Terpinolene has been used as an anti-septic for centuries, and is also anti-bacterial and anti-fungal and is used to treat insomnia in a blend of lilac and lavender.

Therapeutic Benefits of Cannabinoids

CBGA: Analgesic; Anti-inflammatory;

THCA: Anti-cancer; Anti-inflammatory; Anti-spasmodic;

CBDA: Anti-cancer; Anti-inflammatory; **CBCA:** Anti-fungal; Anti-inflammatory;

CBGVA; THCVA; CBDVA; CBCVA and CBNA: Anti-inflammatory;

THC: Analgesic; Anti-bacterial; Anti-cancer; Anti-inflammatory; Anti-spasmodic; Appetite stimulant; Bronchodilator; Neuroprotective;

CBD: Analgesic; Anti-anxiety; Anti-bacterial; Anti-cancer; Anti-convulsive; Anti-depressant; Anti-emetic; Anti-inflammatory; Anti-insomnia; Anti-ischemic; Anti-psychotic; Anti-spasmodic; Bone stimulant; Immunosuppressive; Neuroprotective;

CBC: Analgesic; Anti-bacterial; Anti-cancer; Anti-depressant; Anti-fungal; Anti-inflammatory; Anti-insomnia; Bone stimulant;

CBG: Analgesic; Anti-bacterial; Anti-cancer; Anti-depressant; Anti-fungal; Bone stimulant;

CBN: Analgesic; Anti-bacterial; Anti-convulsive; Anti-inflammatory; Anti-insomnia;

Delta 8-THC: Anti-anxiety; Antiemetic.

Conclusion

After using Rick Simpson Oil (RSO), a DIY cannabis oil that Rick Simpson has shared indiscriminately around the world for those suffering from cancer, I leaned first hand that the cannabis plant is way more valuable than for just recreational use. This book has introduced the reader to testing methods available for identifying and quantifying the cannabinoids in cannabis. In addition, this book reviewed some of the medicinal properties found in the cannabis plant including cannabinoids and terpenes. Not every batch of any given strain of cannabis will contain high levels of terpenes since growing conditions affect the outcome and therefore, it is important to start insisting on a lab analysis that includes not only detected cannabinoids but also detected terpenes.

Using a home testing kit for identifying certain cannabinoids in the Indica strains I am partial to, I was surprised with the outcome of a large presence of CBG and no indication of Cannabidiol (CBD) in any of the three strains tested. Since only "Hot Testing" was performed, it is now understood that the absence of CBD may be due to it evaporating during the heating phase. At the time of testing, the lack of CBD in the test results impelled me to further study the cannabis plant at a deeper level.

The synergy effect of cannabinoids and terpenes offer a great deal of potential benefits which is only beginning to be investigated. As patients become more aware of the complexities in the various compounds found in cannabis, they will become more discerning when choosing the medicine that is right for them. Hopefully, as patients become more aware too, of the full potential of Cannabis preparations, it will help increase the quality of cannabis medications made available to them, along with the quality of information. Educated patients can be the impetus for further research into what can be considered an almost limitless potential for the medical use of cannabis.

Ryder Management Inc

Sample Lab Analysis Reports

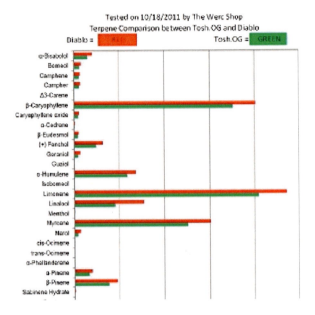

Thewercshop.com

    The above, from The Werc Shop, are examples of lab reports disclosing the breakdown of terpenes in a given sample of cannabis. Information accompanying your medicine that only discloses THC and CBD content can severely skew or limit the benefits of your chosen strain.

A proper profile, such as that shown above, should be available on your chosen strain and should include a complete breakdown of detected cannabinoids and terpenes. Terpenes contain many therapeutic and medicinal benefits that play an important role in your healthcare. It is the synergy effect of all the cannabinoids and terpenes that make this plant based medicine superior to single synthetic molecule therapies manufactured in a lab.

Ryder Management Inc

Know Your Terpenes

TERPENE	BENEFIT	AROMA
Pinene Also found in pine needles	Anti-inflamatory Anti-bacterial Bronchodilator Aids memory	Pine Earth
Myrcene Also found in hops	Sedative Sleep aid Muscle relaxant	Flowers Pungent Earth
Limonene Also found in citrus	Treats acid reflux Anti-anxiety Antidepressant	Citrus Fresh spice
Terpinolene Also found in coriander	Analgesic Pain reduction Digestive aid Stomachic	Pine Herbal Anise Lime
Linalool Also found in lavender	Anesthetic Anti-convulsive Analgesic Anti-anxiety	Flowers Lavender Citrus Fresh spice
Terpineol Also found in mugwort	Calming aid Antibacterial Antiviral Immune system	Pleasant lilac Citrus Wood
Caryophyllene Also found in black pepper	Anti-inflammatory Analgesic Protects cells lining Digestive tract	Citrus Spice
Humulene Also found in basil	Anti-inflamatory	Robust Herbaceous Earth
Ocimene Also found in thyme and alfalfa	Decongestant Antiseptic Antiviral Bactrericidal	Citrusy green Wood Tropical fruit

Other Books by RMI

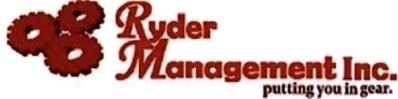

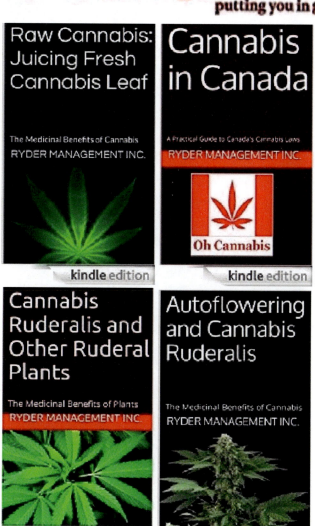

Ryder Management Inc

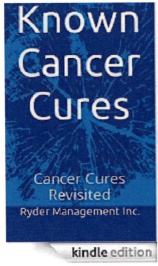
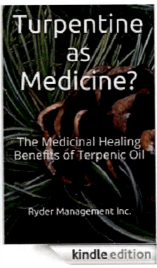
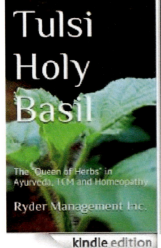
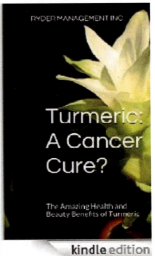

And more …

Ten Native Commandments

1. Treat the Earth and all that dwells therein with respect
2. Remain close to the Great Spirit.
3. Show great respect to your fellow beings.
4. Work together for the benefit of all mankind.
5. Give assistance and kindness wherever needed.
6. Do what you know to be right.
7. Look after the well-being of mind and body.
8. Dedicate a share of your efforts to the greater good.
9. Be truthful and honest at all times.
10. Take full responsibility for your actions.

Made in the USA
San Bernardino, CA
11 July 2015